VAGUS NERVE

BOOK

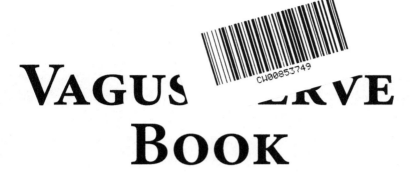

Upgrade your Body's Natural Healing Process through Daily Vagus Nerve Exercises for Controlling Psychiatric and Inflammatory Disorders and Improving Gut-Health

By

Queenie Dillon

DISCLAIMER NOTICE

This book has been independently written and published. Kindly note that the content contained within this publication is provided exclusively for informational and entertainment purposes. Every effort has been made to provide accurate, current, reliable, and complete information. No express or implied assurances are present. The content of this book is intended to aid readers in attaining a more comprehensive understanding of the related subject. The exercises, information, and activities are designed exclusively for self-help. This book does not intend to serve as a substitute for the counsel of professional psychologists, attorneys, financiers, or other experts. Kindly contact a certified professional if you need counseling.

Reading this work, the reader agrees that the author shall not be responsible for any direct or indirect harm caused by the content contained herein, including but not restricted to omissions, errors, or inaccuracies. You are responsible for the decisions, actions, and outcomes that ensue as a reader.

Table of Content

Introduction

So, you have reached this point in life, huh? Don't get me wrong, but this is life. One day, we are absolutely healthy and make the worst decisions in life, and then we reach the point where we simply admit that some things need to be changed.

If you are at the phase of life where you are ready to make some smart decisions and incorporate positive changes in life, you are at the right place! "Vagus Nerve Book" is a complete guide for people who are disturbed because their bodies are not performing optimally or suffering from conditions that affect the Vagus Nerve and thus their health.

If you are wondering now, but what is Vagus Nerve actually? Let me tell you! It is the biggest nerve in the human body that starts from the brain and goes to the intestines. The reason it is least known is because it does not carry out main functions of the body but aids them by communicating with other major organs actively.

I have known and worked with many people who could tell that there was something wrong with their health but they couldn't figure out the reasons. The human body is a complex system that carries out too many functions at a time, making it possible for many people to get confused about whether something is wrong with them or not. But reading this book will bring you one step closer to understanding the underlying connections within the body that shape your present-day choices and actions.

However, you should keep in mind that although this book will teach you all about Vagus Nerves, it is not a replacement for a doctor or medical assistance. If you are experiencing any issues that may or may not be related to Vagus Nerve, getting a full check-up and treatment for it is the first solution, and other interventions are to keep the effects lasting and meaningful.

Become more in-tuned with your body by learning about the vagus nerve, its functions, and specifically how to keep it stimulated to live a relaxed and calm life.

CHAPTER 1

OVERVIEW OF THE "WANDERING NERVE" OF THE BODY

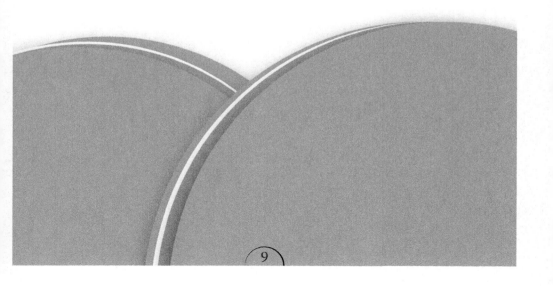

Vagus Nerve has the most curious meaning you could have heard. It literally translates to Wandering Nerve because it is the longest nerve in the body, connecting many organs with the brain to communicate internal and external factors at the same time.

It is part of the parasympathetic nervous system that is responsible for bringing the body back to the resting state after some overdrive.

1.1 Vagus Nerve and Its Purpose

Vagus Nerve can be regarded as the primary communication line between the brain and many organs, such as the heart, lungs, liver, stomach, spleen, kidney, small intestine, and large intestine. It is the 10th cranial nerve that originates from the brain and engages in many important functions.

It passes from the thoracic regions of the brain stem to reach the intestines. It is part of the autonomic nervous system that engages in exchanging sensory information to and from the brain. The brain is responsible for sending only 20% of this sensory information, while the body sends up 80% of this information to the brain for computing.

The name Vagus Nerve may make you think it is just one nerve that travels up and down, but it is actually many nerves joined together to form a complete network. It drops down from both sides of the brain stem to go into different organs and collect sensory information.

1.2 Functions in Body

There are many functions in the body that require assistance from the vagus nerve to complete. They are as follows:

- Muscle and skin sensations such as the outer ear and skin behind the ear.
- It contributes to saliva and mucus production of the body.
- It provides sensory information about the larynx, trachea, and oesophagus, along with aiding in the movement of muscles and subsequent speech.
- It involves itself in mood changes.
- It helps in slowing down the heart rate after the adrenaline rush.
- It performs reflex actions such as swallowing, sneezing, coughing, gagging, or vomiting.
- It controls the blood pressure level.
- It gives taste sensation to the back of the tongue and epiglottis.
- It contributes to breathing and heat regulation of the body.
- It makes involuntary movements in the digestive tract that processes food.

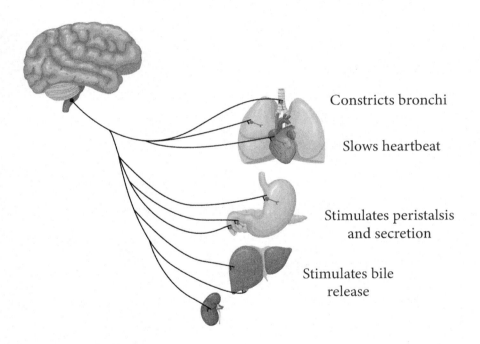

Constricts bronchi

Slows heartbeat

Stimulates peristalsis
and secretion

Stimulates bile
release

1.3 The Gut-Brain Axis

The Gut-Brain Axis, as we have discussed before, the to-and-fro motion of the information happens in a body constantly. The brain analyzes situations and gives commands to all organs to prepare for the situation the body is facing.

Similarly, the organs send their own reports to the brain to adapt accordingly. The nexus keeps working together to help the body at all times. The results depend entirely on what a person faces, positive or negative, but a solution is always presented.

In this Gut-Brain Axis, microbiota plays the most crucial role. It is responsible for the bidirectional interactions between the gut and the brain. Each person hosts trillions of microbiotas (communities of microbes) in various parts of the body.

When talking about the relationship between the gut and the brain, these microbiota work in unison with the brain to carry out daily functions of the digestive tract by communicating any possible changes in real-time. All of this process is supported and runs through the vagus nerve, which carries the sensory information and relays it to the brain.

1.4 Sympathetic and Parasympathetic Nervous System

All involuntary functions and actions that are carried out by our brain are conducted through the autonomic nervous system. This autonomic nervous system is split into two branches: the sympathetic nervous system and the parasympathetic nervous system.

Sympathetic Nervous System is responsible for the "fight or flight" response of the body in a stressful or sudden situation. It prepares the body for intense events that need immediate intervention.

The Parasympathetic Nervous System is responsible for bringing the body back after a sudden adrenaline rush. It focuses on bringing the body to "rest and digest" mode that neutralizes the consequences of being in a state of high alert.

Both sympathetic and parasympathetic nervous systems are sides of the same coin: your body. They work in contrast to each other to always keep your bodily functions in tune with each other.

Did You Know?

About 75% of the parasympathetic nervous system consists of vagal nerves.

CHAPTER 2

POLYVAGAL THEORY

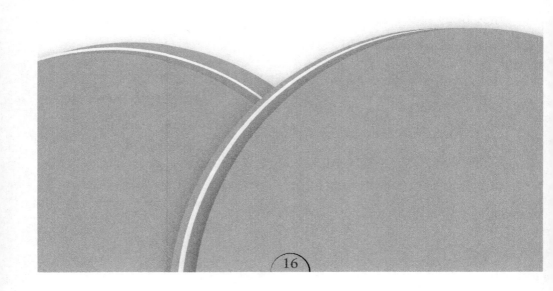

Humans need a safe environment to live well and thrive. That feeling of safety is also our normal rest mode that our bodies function on. Polyvagal theory is based on finding the cause of those feelings of safety that help us relax and not keep us looking over our shoulders all the time. Dr. Stephen Porges proposed the polyvagal theory to go into the details of how a person goes through physical and psychological changes when in-between situations arise that require the body to either go into overdrive or pull back into a resting state.

2.1 The Concept of Neuroception

Sensing danger is one of the most basic characteristics that humans and animals share. Every animal can take cues from the environment to deem it safe or unsafe. This process of percepting the environment and behaving accordingly is called neuroception by Dr. Stephen.

In neuroception, you take in your surroundings by scanning around involuntarily and acting according to your perceived notions. If you enter a room at your house, you may take a quick look and relax as your neural transmitters send the message that everything is alright. In the same way, if you enter that same room and find some of your items stolen, you will immediately perceive it as a threat and act accordingly.

This process of neuroception works through the vagus nerve, which is responsible for communicating this information between the brain and the organs. A vagus nerve is stimulated on both sides (ventral and dorsal), and the most interesting fact is that the ventral side handles cues related to safety in interactions and environments while the dorsal side works with cues of danger.

Three Stages of Response

Our responses are instantaneous; we never wait to respond to any situation that needs an immediate reaction. However, according to Dr. Porges, evolution has played a vital part in the development of responses over decades and centuries and in the events that the human race has faced. He speculates that our responses have gone through three developmental stages to reach this point in history and time. They include:

- Immobilization
- Mobilization
- Social Engagement

Immobilization

Immobilization is termed as the oldest response pathway. It occurs when a person senses extreme danger and decides to stay still in response. The responses that can be put in this category are being numb, completely frozen, or shutting down as a response.

Mobilization

According to Dr. Porges, our responses to threat were modified as part of evolution. From immobilization, we moved toward mobilization, where a person sprang into action in the face of danger instead of freezing up. It happens when you get an adrenaline rush to perform a "fight or flight" response to a threat.

Social Engagement

Social engagement is the latest addition in the hierarchy of responses. It stimulates the ventral vagus nerve, which makes you feel safe and connected, providing a sense of security and calmness through engagement with others.

Now, we may assume that these responses are rigid and that only one can be selected, but the truth is that we can easily practice any number of responses at any time. For example, upon getting caught for doing something naughty, a child may freeze for a second or two before running away in fear of getting scolded.

In the same way, any person can demonstrate any or all responses one by one. Once you understand these key points that trigger your responses, you can deal with things and responses that you may display in your daily life.

Get in the habit of observing your own actions and try to be mindful about pointing out the thoughts and measures that are triggered by your vagus nerve, too.

CHAPTER 3

DYSFUNCTION IN VAGUS NERVE

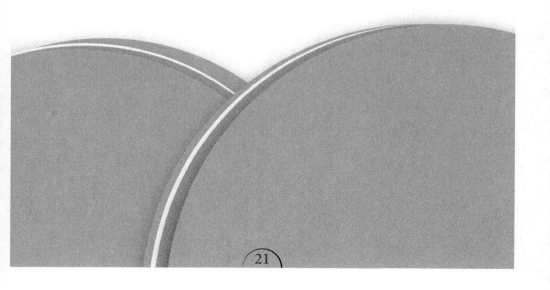

Dysfunction in the vagus nerve occurs when it gets inflamed or infected for a number of reasons. Experiencing mental or physical stress for longer periods of time can also damage the vagus nerve.

This damage may include:

- Problems in swallowing
- Loss of voice or hoarseness in it
- Acid Reflux
- Dizziness spells
- Abnormal positioning of Uvula
- Sudden weight loss or obesity
- Inactive gag reflex
- Abdominal pain or bloating
- Nausea or vomiting
- Inflammatory issues
- Gastrointestinal issues
- Cardiovascular issues

Apart from the suggestions provided in the list, there can be some other reasons of dysfunction in the vagus nerve as well. There are some disorders that can also affect the vagus nerve. We will discuss all possibilities in this chapter ahead.

3.1 Testing for Vagal Dysfunction

Vagal Nerve may not be a popular test subject in the medical field, but every day, new theories are tested, and new ways are being discovered that help you reach the root cause in a better manner.

The tests we are discussing here are the ones that are great for overall usage by common people without subjecting themselves to any harm. Once you perform these tests, feel reassured by getting good results or make a plan with permission from your doctor to lead yourself towards a better life.

The Wrist Pulse Test

For the Wrist Pulse Test, you need to follow these steps:

- Put your index finger on your wrist and feel the pulse.
- Track the rhythm before taking a deep breath and pay attention to the beats while you are breathing in and out.

The in-breaths should have less time interval between the pulses than the out-breaths. The beats should be stronger and faster while breathing in and slow and less in breathing out. If your result is similar to the described outcome, it means that your ventral vagal function is all right and completely healthy.

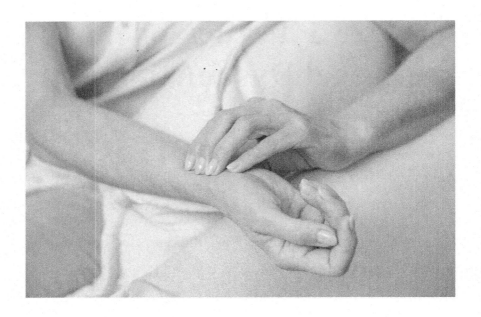

Uvula Deviation Testing

For this test, you need a partner to perform the check-up since you cannot do it yourself. The steps are as follows:

- Ask your partner to grab a torch or flashlight.
- Sit in a comfortable position and open your mouth wide so that the partner can examine the uvula.
- Once the partner tells you that they can see the uvula, start producing an "Ah, Ah!" sound. The partner may use a tongue depressor to see the back of the throat more clearly.
- Ask them to observe the uvula and tell if the uvula moves to one side while producing the sound.

If there is no deviation in the uvula, it means the vagus nerve is healthy as it should be, and if there is deviation, visit a doctor for a thorough check-up.

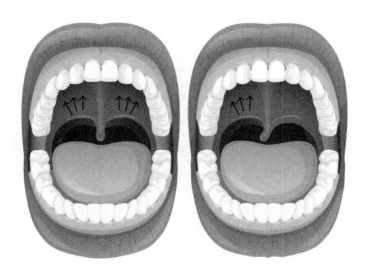

Speech and Noise Test

In the Speech and Noise Test, the focus is on noticing the abnormalities in the voice after swallowing water. This test also requires help from a partner to look for minute details that may not be noticed otherwise. Here is what you need to do:

- Ask your partner to sit beside you.
- Take a big gulp of water, swallow it, and start talking.
- Ask them to look for signs of hoarseness, whispering, nasal tone, or regurgitation of liquid from the nose.

If any of the symptoms are noticed, consult a doctor for a proper follow-up.

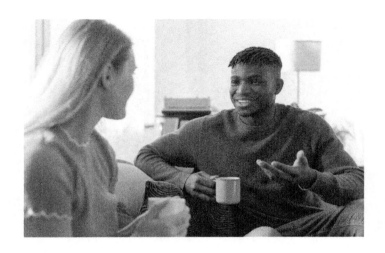

The Shoulder Squeeze Test

In the Shoulder Squeeze Test, you need to follow these steps:

- Use your thumb and index finger to lightly squeeze the trapezius muscle on each of your shoulders.

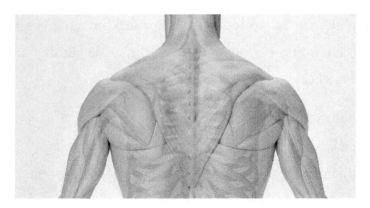

Trapezius Muscle

- Compare both muscles in terms of softness to hardness level. A healthy and stress-free trapezius muscle should be soft and elastic to the touch. If one or both sides are hard, do the Trapezius Muscle exercise that is provided on page 46.

Gag Reflex Test

This test must be performed by a trained doctor or physician. Do not attempt yourself or with a partner who may not understand the consequences.

In this test, the doctor will test your gag reflex, which stops foreign objects from going into your throat. The steps are as follows:

- In the examination, the doctor will use a tongue depressor to keep the tongue down and use a cotton swab to touch the inner walls of the throat.
- The action will make you gag, so try to keep yourself calm and poised.
- If you do not feel the need to gag, it means that the vagus nerve is damaged.

3.2 Disorders or Issues Linked to Vagus Nerve

Once you have tested your reflexes, it is better to educate yourself on the disorders that are related to the vagus nerve. If any of these issues rings a bell, it is better to stay prepared rather than letting yourself go haywire over it. In this section, let's go over such issues in detail:

Disorders Caused by Vagus Nerve

The vagus nerve may play an important role in the body, but like all other parts, it can also cause a number of issues once it gets damaged or disrupted from its duties. The vagus nerve, however, is just a communicator between the organs and does not operate on different multitudes. For this reason, the complications that it can cause in the body are also limited. Let's look at them here:

Vasovagal Syncope

Vasovagal syncope occurs when a person experiences harsh or sudden effects of situations because of vagus nerve overdrive. The causes could include pain, anxiety, stress, hunger, or extreme heat. It happens when the blood pressure drops too quickly for the body to be able to regulate it easily. A person may feel dizzy or faint as a result of vasovagal syncope.

Gastroparesis

Gastroparesis is a condition in which a damaged vagus nerve does not allow the stomach to completely pass on food to the intestines. This condition can develop after abdominal surgery, from diabetes, or a viral infection.

There are a few symptoms that may indicate gastroparesis:

- Acid reflux
- Pain or bloating in the abdominal area
- Vomiting or nausea
- Feeling full as soon as starting a meal
- Constant fluctuation in blood sugar levels
- Weight loss

Consult with a doctor if and when you start experiencing these symptoms simultaneously.

Disorders That May Need Vagus Nerve Reset to Heal

Some disorders that occur in the body need interventions of some sort. One of these interventions may be the vagus nerve reset.

Vagus nerve reset can be carried out by the VNS device that keeps the body working properly.

Role of Vagus Nerve Stimulation (VNS)

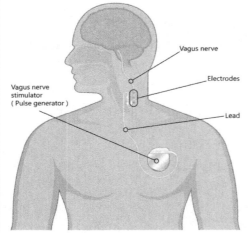

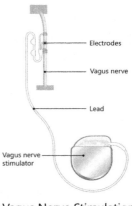

Vagus Nerve Stimulation
(VNS)

VNS Device

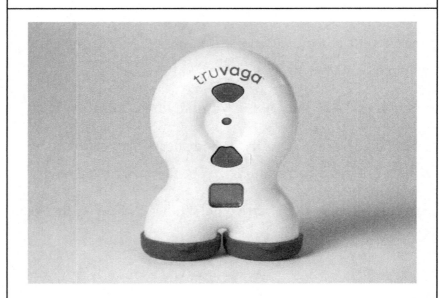

Hand-held Stimulator

Vagus Nerve Stimulator (VNS) is a small device that sends mild to low pulses to the brain stem by stimulating the vagus nerve. It is akin to a pacemaker, but instead of aiding the heart in its function, VNS helps the brain by sending signals that change brain cells accordingly.

Once these charges are received in the brain stem, they are disseminated to the targeted organ(s) connected through the vagus nerve. Although it may seem like a viable option, there is not enough research on its usage to be used widely.

In most cases, it is used as a last resort to help patients who develop treatment resistance and experience worse symptoms than the average patients. It is most commonly used to treat patients with chronic epilepsy, depression, and stroke. But it is not for pregnant women or people with breathing problems or heart arrhythmia.

Let's find out how vagus nerve stimulation can play a role in the management of these chronic illnesses.

Depression

Severe and persistent depression that keeps coming back or doesn't respond to any number of treatments is given the last resort to use VNS for treatment.

The VNS helps jolt the vagus nerve to improve the overall mood.

Chronic Epilepsy

Most epilepsy patients can control themselves with the help of medication. However, there is a small percentage of patients who require VNS as an additional measure to control focal seizures.

Heart Stroke

For heart stroke patients, VNS is considered as an additional rehabilitation method that focuses on opening blocked arteries. It helps in clearing up moderate to severe loss of function in the hands and arms.

Rheumatoid Arthritis

Rheumatoid arthritis is a severe anti-inflammatory issue that causes swelling and pain in the joints. Recent studies have shown that VNS can reduce the severity of RA in chronic patients.

Inflammatory Bowel Disease (IBD)

Inflammatory bowel disease is another serious disease that causes inflammation in the GI tract of the body. It is a life-long disease that can be managed but there is no permanent cure to this day. Vagus nerve stimulation is currently being tested for IBD patients to offer them temporary relief from pain.

It is said to be a disorder related to the imbalance of the autonomous nervous system that the VNS may be able to regulate for the most part, relieving the patients from experiencing any extreme symptoms and taking them towards bearable pain and other side effects.

CHAPTER 4

PHYSICAL EXERCISES
FOR RELAXATION

Physical exercise plays the most important role in fostering a healthy lifestyle. Any person who does not take measures to stay fit cannot enjoy a happy life for long. If you are one of those people who do not bother with including a physical fitness routine, it may be your time to start now.

The first tip we can give to a beginner is to start slowly. Starting a 5-minute workout routine to going up to 30 or 40 minutes should take gradual time that allows a person to adjust well with the exercises.

Once you have tried a number of exercises, you can easily pick out the ones that have proven most beneficial to you and keep repeating them in your daily routine. Nothing works better than the mindset that everything is achievable with a little bit of hard work and resilience.

Follow the exercises provided ahead to relax your mind and body.

Stimulation Exercise

One exercise to stimulate your vagus nerve is as follows:

- Lie down on the ground and interlace your finger behind the head. The fingers should be at the base of the skull.

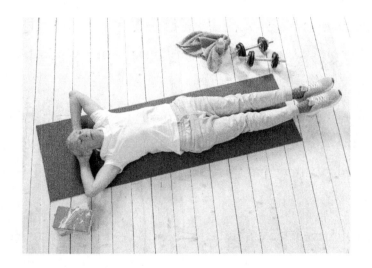

- Do not move your head and look to the right with your eyes. While looking, sigh, swallow, and yawn.
- Now repeat the same step on the left side.

You can blink in-between the exercise but do not move your head or eyes while performing it. You can also re-take the vagal nerve test to see if there are any changes.

Stretching

Stretches can be of many kinds, featuring all parts of the body. You need to exercise your neck to stimulate the vagus nerve through the workout.

In Figure 1, you can see the restive pose you need to make. The steps are as follows:

- First, tilt your head toward the left direction. While doing so, keep a little pressure on the head through the left hand. Once you get in the pose, stare 5 seconds into the opposite direction by simply moving the eyes.
- Now repeat the same step on the other side and complete the whole set 3 more times.

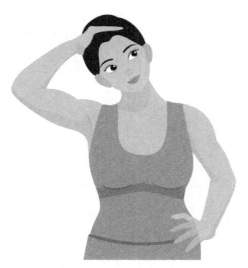

Figure 1

For the Figure 2, take the following steps:

- Repeat the instructions from the previous set while simply adding the other hand's position into the exercise. By keeping the other hand, repeat the same sets as before (3 times).
- Also, note that you may feel a yawn coming in; it is because of the exercise. If your parasympathetic system is activated, you are likelier to experience such results in between.

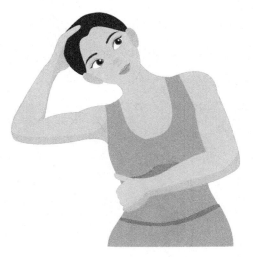

Figure 2

Yoga

Practicing yoga has gained popularity in the last few years. It is the best way to train your body to exert force yet stay calm and relaxed, especially in today's busy world. Among the number of benefits yoga has, increasing vagal tone is one of them.

You can choose to get into yoga by taking proper classes or learning from online videos and sessions simply to avail yourself of its numerous benefits. But if you are looking to specifically learn poses that are best for vagus nerve stimulation, they are as follows in a complete sequence:

Meditative Sitting Pose

- Start the yoga exercise with an easy pose to ease into the routine by sitting down on a yoga mat and folding your legs.
- Now, put your shoulders straight by relaxing the body.
- Put one hand on your belly and the other in the lap before taking a deep breath from the diaphragm. When you inhale, your belly should press into your hand.
- Keep taking deep breaths for at least 5-10 minutes that engage the belly while focusing on the sensation you feel in the body.
- If your mind keeps wandering, gently pull your focus back to the exercise at hand.
- When you are done, blink your eyes open and take time to return to the present.

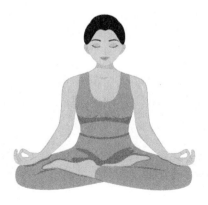

Cat-Cow Pose

- Take a position on all fours.
- Your wrists should be in line with the shoulders, and knees in line with the hips. Balance your weight before starting the exercise.
- Go into the pose by first breathing in and then tilting your face upwards. Your stomach should drop down towards the mat.
- Now, breathe out before pulling your chin into the chest.
- Try bringing your navel towards the spine, making it arch, as shown in the picture.
- Be completely focused on the pose while doing it, and focus on releasing the tension.
- Hold the pose for 60 seconds before resting.

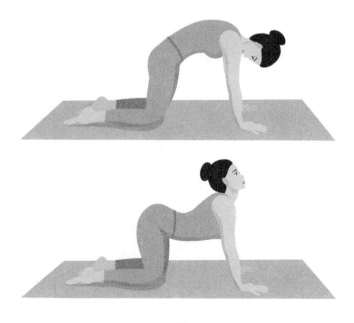

Forward Fold Pose

- Again, get on all fours while aligning wrists with shoulders and knees with the hips.
- Press into the hands to support the body while you tuck the toes and lift the knees.
- Slowly bring your hips up until the body starts making an inverted "V" shape.
- To move into the correct posture, bend the knees slightly while lengthening the spine and tailbone.
- Getting into the position, your heels should automatically be slightly raised from the ground.
- If you feel imbalanced, press into the hands and distribute the weight.
- The head must stay in line with the upper arms, and the chin should be tucked in.
- Once you are in the pose, hold it for 60 seconds before releasing the body gently.

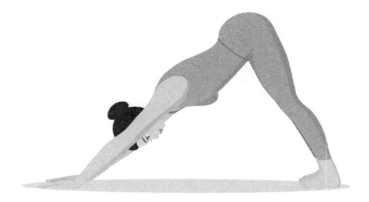

Child's Pose

- For the child's pose, sit on the mat by first kneeling on the knees and folding the legs underneath. Your buttocks should rest on your heels. It will stretch your thigh muscles.
- Now lean forward while letting the legs stay folded in their place and placing the forehead on the mat.
- Extend your arms in front of you on both sides of the head and keep them slightly stretched.
- Try deep breathing while staying in the pose.
- Keep inhaling and exhaling for 60 seconds before resting.

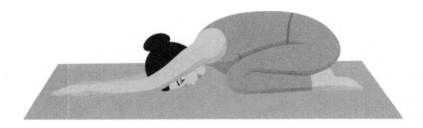

Waterfall Pose

*For this exercise, you need a block or sturdy box
that can bear weight.*

- Lie down on the mat and place the block under the tailbone.
- Slightly bend the knees before lifting the feet in the air. Take your time and slowly get into the pose.
- Let the muscles relax as you feel the gravity sinking you into the ground.

- Rotate the feet in circles while taking ten deep breaths.
- Once done, break the pose by gently bringing your legs down and resting for a few moments.

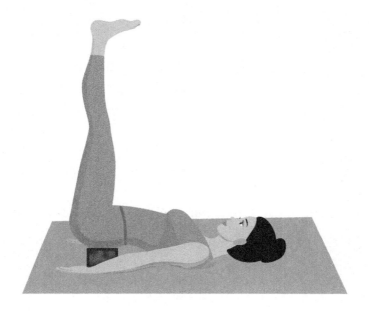

Corpse Pose

- In this last pose, bring your body into a relaxed state by lying down and extending your arms and legs.
- Breathe in from the nose and breathe out from the mouth.
- Do not try to control your breathing or actions, and simply allow yourself to release the body's tension through your breaths.
- Practice breathing for 60 seconds before letting yourself simply rest in the pose and taking in the after-effects.

- Get up and going when you have returned to the present and worn off the tiredness of the body.

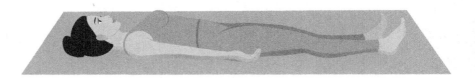

Vagal Push

The vagal push is an exercise that can force your vagal nerve to regulate by giving internal pushes that open up your body circulations from the inside. Never try to perform the push while you are sitting or standing. It may cause you to faint or feel lightheaded.

For this exercise, perform the steps as follows:

- Lie down on your back.
- Tense up the muscles in the abdomen and push internally as you do for bowel movement.
- Keep holding your breath while performing the previous step for about 15 to 20 seconds.
- Take a break and repeat the same steps 3 to 4 more times. Ideally, the break could be up to 2 minutes.

This exercise will stimulate your vagus nerves, and it is also a very helpful way of controlling fast heart rhythm, which is difficult to control otherwise.

Daily Exercise in any Form or Sports

Staying fit has never cost anyone. If you are looking forward to getting positive results in physical or mental health, start incorporating exercise into your daily routine. Although gyms are a great source of dedicated motivation, they are not optimal for all.

If you are also one of those people who excel outside the mandated environment, look for sports or exercises that grab your interest. You may start walking, cycling, running, swimming, hiking, or any other type of activity that can motivate you to keep going every day without feeling too burdened.

You may also play games such as football, basketball, soccer, baseball, or any other one to become an active person in general.

Cold Exposure

Extreme cold can give you a jump start whenever you are in need of a boost. Have you ever had a friend or sibling who loves to sneak up on you to touch your face with cold hands when you are feeling completely cozy and warm? This same example works very well here.

You can reset your vagus nerve by experiencing cold and rewiring yourself to get back to the original state of ease after a flight or fight response.

In cold exposure, you can simply dip your hand or face in ice-cold water or take a short cold shower. Similarly, you can also wear fewer layers of clothes to let yourself feel the natural cold.

Exposure should be timed and can be started with 30 seconds that is increased gradually. Regular exposure can help you condition yourself to relax more and create a long-lasting positive change.

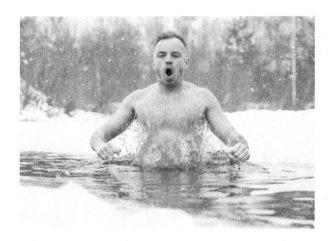

Trapezius Muscle Stimulation

When you do the shoulder squeeze test and feel that the shoulders are tense, do this stimulation exercise to activate the vagal nerve and release the tension that is stored there. You can do this by taking the following steps:

- Sit down in a comfortable seat with a straight back.
- Use your left hand to squeeze the right shoulder for around 10 to 20 seconds and yawn, sigh, and swallow.

- Now, repeat the same step on the left shoulder.
- Take a break and repeat the same steps again if you feel the need.

You can easily spend 2 minutes each day performing this basic exercise.

Laughing Exercise

Laughing is an action that helps you in countless ways. It reduces stress, boosts a good mood, stimulates the vagal nerve, and strengthens your immune system. When stuck in negative and stressful situations, it is best to stay calm and force yourself to feel better by laughing heartily.

You may use a little help by watching a funny video or show that can make you laugh or try a laughter therapy session to have an interactive way of dispelling the negative that is affecting your body.

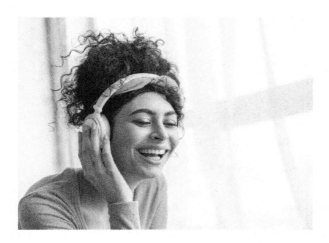

Gargling Practice

Gargling may sound like an odd choice when our concern is the vagus nerve, but it makes complete sense. When we gargle, we hear our voice. It is because the vocal cords are engaged in gargling. The back of the throat, as well as vocal cords, are attached to the vagus nerve, and they can help in its activation.

So, add gargling to your daily exercise routine. Even 10 seconds in the morning or night routine can prove to be very beneficial.

Singing and Humming

As we discussed just now, the vocal cords are directly connected to the vagal nerve. Using your voice to sing or hum for a while can help you exercise the nerves.

It is a very easy practice that you can also enjoy practicing (if your voice is good; if not, practice might make it better, right?). So, include singing and humming at least one song daily into your routine.

Chanting

It may be similar to singing and humming in terms of the use of muscles and the benefits produced, but chanting is another way to exercise the vocal cords as well as the vagus nerve.

Chanting daily for 5 minutes can be easily incorporated into your routine without disrupting the flow. Have you ever heard or seen the Hindu practice of chanting 'Om' while meditating? It can be taken as the perfect example.

In the same way, you can practice chanting long 'Om' sounds while listening to the vibrations around the ears.

Dancing

Dancing is another great physical activity that gives you room to enjoy yourself while healing yourself from the inside. Many adults are not in tune with their bodies because of letting go of exercise in life.

Dancing is a form of exercise that can help you express yourself. If you feel shy, you may practice dancing alone, but if you tend to thrive in social situations, plan frequent get-togethers where everyone can dance and enjoy.

Zumba Exercise

Zumba exercise is an amalgamation of dance and aerobic exercise that puts moving around at the forefront. Although it is most popular for weight loss and general activity, the vagus nerve can be stimulated by it as well.

If you are searching for a fun and easy way to keep yourself healthy, attending Zumba classes (online or offline) can also help you stay true to your goal of stimulating the vagus nerve.

Acupuncture

Acupuncture is one of the ancient Chinese remedies for optimizing a body's functioning. There are many acupuncture points on the body that can increase vagal activity substantially after the interaction. Each acupuncture point carries its own significance, but you should be careful about approaching experienced personnel only.

A trained acupuncturist can easily give you a personalized treatment that your body severely needs to feel refreshed and anew. Make an appointment with someone who knows the craft well, and you may choose to add it to your monthly routine if it helps.

Getting a Massage

Massage is an easy yet effective method to not only relax your mind and body but also to decrease the activity level of the vagus nerve. Each body part can feel ease and relief after massage, improving overall condition of the body but vagus nerve stimulation can be achieved by massaging the scalp, ears, or feet.

Out of the massage able areas for vagus nerve stimulation, feet need a good reflexology session to properly induce the good sensations that regulate the vagus nerve. For ear-based stimulation, follow the method described ahead.

- Put your index finger in your upper ear in the ridge (triangular fossa) and lightly rotate your finger to massage the area.

- Massage the area for around 10 to 30 seconds or until you feel a sense of calm.

TIP!

Massage both ears at the same time to get maximum benefit out of it.

- In the next step, put your index finger in the ear canal and press it towards the back before making gentle circles on the area. Keep lightly massaging the place for about 10 to 30 seconds.
- To check if the ear has loosened, pull your ears and note if they feel tightened or not. If yes, then repeat the exercises, and if not, then stop the exercise and try again when you feel the need to stimulate the vagus nerve again.

Neck Massage for Carotid Artery

Out of all functions of the vagus nerve, running the carotid artery is one of the main responsibilities. When the body refuses to return to its normal functioning, you can use this technique to bring it back. This way, you can slow down the heart rate and allow it to climb down from the high work pace that it was forced to work on. Here is how you can perform this massage:

- Lie down on your back.
- Turn your head to one side.
- Take your hand to the carotid artery and feel the pulse.
- Where the pulse is at its strongest, gently massage the area in longitudinal strides for 5 - 10 seconds.

- Stop the massage and see if the heart rate is normalizing. If not, try the exercise again in a minute or perform the same steps on the other side of the neck.

By following this method, the increased heat rate should come back to its normal pace. If not, visit a doctor for a detailed check-up.

Playing Wind Instruments

Playing Wind Instruments such as the flute or kazoo can help you stretch your vocal cords, and, in turn, the vagus nerve relieves itself of tension and gives you time to manage your physical stresses in a better way.

One Favorite Activity a Day

The vagus nerve is targeted not only directly but also indirectly. If you can give yourself some time each day to enjoy something you love or enjoy, it will bring you many benefits. A simple stroll in the park or beach, watching a sunset, or eating a favorite food can help you and your body relax.

Make time for yourself to enjoy one thing each day, no matter how small, and give your body resting time after a stressful day of work or an issue at home. It will help you unwind and have some downtime.

Take a Reflexology Session

Reflexology is an aspect of massage therapy that focuses on working with hands, feet, and neck pressure points to heal the body from the inside. These pressure points stimulate organs that are connected via the vagus nerve.

These organs get a boost through external points that allow them to stimulate the vagus nerve. Reflexology also works on bringing these major organs to rest mode by resetting the vagus nerve whenever needed. It reduces pain, stress, and anxiety while improving your mood and general well-being.

Forest Bathing

Forest bathing is an activity that works for anyone looking for a change of pace from their busy and hectic lives. If you find it difficult to slide into your resting mode for the betterment of the body, try looking for a forest bathing place around your town.

It may sound difficult, but it is simply the inclusion of natural scenery in your daily life. Spending time in a forest will help you improve your mood, release stress, and stimulate the vagus nerve.

If you are not close to such a place that offers such services, you can also go to a place that is filled with greenery and offers a stimulating yet relaxing environment. A 20-minute stroll around a nice, quiet place can help you feel much better.

Biofeedback Check

Biofeedback is the way a doctor measures your nervous system's working output. It can also be used to train the nervous system, but an important tip is to not try this exercise by yourself and wait for a doctor to suggest it according to your symptoms.

Nonetheless, it is the best way to give feedback in a timely and accurate manner that a doctor gets directly from the body.

In biofeedback, a person is monitored with changes in breathing patterns, heart rate, muscle movement, and brain activity. Based on the results, a doctor makes observations and suggestions that can help you go towards a better lifestyle.

Play with a Pet

Playing with a pet that is near and dear to your heart can also help you relax and unwind in a calm environment. Positive interaction with pets can stimulate vagus nerves, allowing the body to calm down by feeling a sense of ease and comforted by the familiar presences that carry the essence of home.

Pets also provide a sense of safety that can allow you to return to being your usual self. There is no limit on interactions or playing time with pets; you may spend any amount of time each day that makes you feel relaxed and happy at home.

4.1 Benefits of Using Exercises to Reset the Vagus Nerve

Exercise has numerous benefits for your health. If you ever feel down or out of sorts, a good physical workout can release the endorphins in the body while the mental exercises focus on bringing peace and calm to your head.

The feelings that you experience are channeled to your brain via the vagus nerve; they chain the positive and negative aspects of your feelings and keep the brain in a constant loop with all other interconnected parts of the body.

In terms of benefits, vagus nerve stimulation exercises help with:

Vagal Tone

The exercises ensure that stresses of the body do not affect the vagus nerve or hinder its function. The exercises allow you to bounce back from negative situations that you surely face in life in one way or another.

Improves Digestion

Performing vagal nerve exercises can have a positive effect on the digestive system of the body. It reduces the effects of bloating, indigestion, or other symptoms of digestion-related issues such as IBS.

A stimulated vagus nerve supports the increase of gastric acid as well as nutrition absorption in the digestive function of the body.

Reducing Anxiety

Anxiety can be a nerve-wracking feeling that makes a person feel helpless in extremely worrisome situations. By performing mental and physical exercises, you can train yourself to calm down in times of high stress levels and improve your mood and body subsequently.

Better Sleep

Practicing exercises such as stretching before going to bed can help stimulate the vagus nerve. It can help improve mood and sleep quality.

A good night's sleep can prepare you for a healthy and fresh day afterward.

Reducing Inflammation

The vagus nerve also plays a role in the management of inflammation in the organs that are connected through it. It is being studied as a part of the treatment, and it suggests that vagal activity helps reduce inflammation as well as the risks of inflammation-related diseases. This is the reason it is producing positive results in the treatment of inflammatory bowel disease (IBD) and rheumatoid arthritis.

Migraine Relief

Migraine is known for being the most severe type of headache. It presents itself in the half-head area while also increasing the person's light and sound sensitivity. Using vagal nerve exercises can allow you to feel relief sooner because it can engage and calm the parasympathetic nervous system, soothing the intense pain of migraine.

CHAPTER 5

MENTAL EXERCISES TO UNWIND THE STRESS

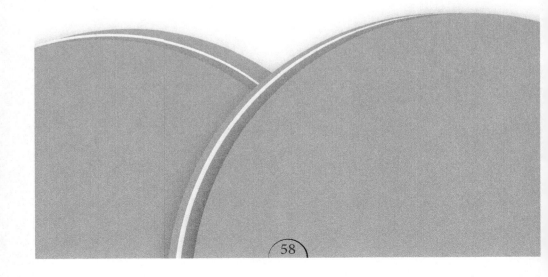

Vagus nerve stimulation is not only done with the help of physical exercises but also with mental exercises. When you need a mental break from the stresses of the world, perform the exercises that we will discuss ahead to keep yourself in a relaxed state of mind.

The exercises will help you release stress and anxiety, as well as build emotional and mental capacity to endure difficult situations in the future.

Finding and Moving on from Triggers

Thinking, or even overthinking, can prove to be too much for most people. They abstain from replaying their thoughts, actions, or events over and over in the head, positive or negative, to analyze what they could have done better.

Instead of running away from anything that causes you grief, the best bet is to sit in a comfortable spot or lie down under a warm weighted blanket and access your triggers. Think about what sets you off, which things you experienced in a day that could have been dealt better, and other such questions that can lead you closer to finding the cause.

The goal of this exercise is not to judge yourself; rather, to make peace with things that can throw your mind and body off balance with pressure. Such introspection each day, even for 10 minutes at a time, can bring you towards acceptance of yourself, calming your mind and body.

Listening to Relaxing and Calm Music

Music has been known to produce soothing effects on the mind. The vagus nerve is also stimulated by music, which helps with focus and promotes the activation of the parasympathetic nervous system.

It helps in producing a calming and relaxing effect that generates happiness. Listening to music helps anyone in transitioning from an intense situation to the restive mode, which also boosts mental clarity and stamina.

Making a Gratitude Journal

Expressing gratitude and being thankful is the best way of relaxing and making yourself feel at ease. Using narrative writing can help you raise your heart rate variability, lower heart rate and stress, as well as strengthen the immune system. All of these things help the vagus nerve keep working appropriately.

So, use this technique to pen down your thoughts and feelings regarding what you faced in a day, what happened, how it happened, and what you can do next time so as not to face any adverse effects in the future.

Challenging events or situations have many layers to the stories. No one goes on to burst at the people out of anger for no reason. Taking time to analyze your actions and ideas can help you feel thankful for each little blessing.

Saying and Believing Positive Affirmations

Affirmation is anything that brings inner peace to you and has a soothing effect on your usual nervous self. Most of the time, we take on more responsibilities and stress than we can shoulder. We keep digging our own grave by adding more and more till the body itself starts exhibiting signs of damage.

In terms of mental assurance and self-soothing attitude, making and saying small yet meaningful phrases to yourself can have an incredible impact on your life. Make up positive affirmations like, "I am healthy," "I am happy," "I am resourceful," or other such phrases that carry deep and meaningful wisdom that you wish to abide by and experience the magic of words.

Take 5 minutes out of your morning routine to give yourself a mental boost of confidence and love. Believe that the words will bring positive change to you, and keep practicing until it actually does.

Deep Breathing Exercise

Deep breathing is an exercise that may help you stimulate the vagus nerve, but it works well for rejuvenating the body and mind in intense situations. No matter what you are going through, breathing deeply can create a way to expel the worries along with the air.

Here is how you can use the 4-7-8 technique to breathe deeply:

- Sit in a comfortable chair that supports your back. Put the tongue on the upper part of the mouth and exhale completely.
- Take four seconds to inhale the air through the nose. Try to engage your diaphragm rather than the chest cavity in the whole exercise.

- Hold your breath inside for seven seconds before expelling the air through the rounded mouth in an audible manner. Take eight seconds to exhale calmly.

All of the steps until now make up one complete round. Repeat the steps in the same order until you feel any physiological changes in your body.

Try to start with 4-5 rounds and adjust the numbers according to the effects and benefits it provides for you.

Sleeping

Sleep is an important factor that many of us often compromise on. Getting 7 to 9 hours of uninterrupted sleep can not only help you stay fresh but also bring out positive changes in your overall mood, health, and patience level.

When you sleep, the body takes that time to cleanse out the toxins that can inflict harm. It helps with repairing and resting, making efforts to stay up-to-date and ready to fight. Try to get recommended hours of sleep to regulate your vagus nerve function as well as other important ones.

Lying Down on the Right Side

Lying down on your right side has many benefits. It allows the body to stay functional without pressing or pressuring any organ more than necessary. It also allows the heart to slow down while sleeping and keep circulating the blood in the most optimal way.

Here is how you can correct your own posture for lying down:

- Lie down on the bed and turn to the right side. Put your head on the pillow to support the neck.
- Make sure that the shoulders are aligned with each other and their center is in line with the chin and center of the hips.
- Keep the head straight in the right direction; it should not be tilted or twisted.
- Make sure the hands and arms are aligned. You may keep them straight on the sides or ahead of you.
- If your hips or knees feel uncomfortable in the position, keep a pillow or a cushion between the knees to provide additional support.

This position is best for anyone who wishes to keep the vagal nerves healthy by maintaining a good posture that relieves other issues, such as breathing issues or pain in various parts of the body.

Eye Movement Exercise

Our eyes tend to revolve around, always looking for something, warning of dangers, and helping us perform each and every task, no matter how minuscule. Flitting around may have numerous uses, but at the same time, they are one of the most overlooked organs of our body. Our eyes are linked to our brains, and sometimes they get tired, too. It is best to keep exercising eye movements to keep them (and the brain) in good shape, too.

Here is what you will have to do:

- Pick any small item, such as a piece of paper or a keychain, and hold it in front of your face.
- The item should be at least four or more inches away from the face. Stare at the object for twenty seconds.
- After the time is up, look far off into the distance and find any object to focus on for another twenty seconds.
- Repeat the steps in a cyclic manner for about four or five times more.
- Once done, relax your eyes slowly and close them to rest for a few seconds before resuming your usual routine.

Socializing in a Relaxing Environment

Humans are social animals. They thrive on finding connections and building relationships with others. Having family and friends can have many benefits for a person, but if the interactions are positive and uplifting, the number of benefits increases tenfold.

Talking about the vagus nerve specifically, positive social interactions help it by improving the vagal tone, positive emotions, and overall mood. It also helps by reducing anxiety and stress in humans.

If you can count on even a single person to improve your state of mind, talk and socialize with them regularly to expel the frustrations from the body and let positive emotions embrace you.

Praying

Praying may seem like an odd choice to most people, but it is a proven way of increasing vagal activity in the body. The rosary prayer, more specifically, is deemed most helpful because it allows you to complete cycles of prayer and regulate your breathing.

You may notice that when you are praying on the rosary, the number of seconds you take to complete the prayer is the same interval you take to breathe. Thus regulating the function without your knowledge!

It increases the HRV (Heart Rate Variability) and vagal function and enhances the heart rhythm, which keeps your body working correctly at all times.

Touch and Vibration Therapy Devices

Suppose personal interventions do not prove very helpful. In that case, you can also choose to go on another route and buy a therapy device that uses sensations of touch and vibration to relay the message to the body that it is in a safe and controlled environment where it can stop overworking itself and go into the rest and digest mode.

Such devices are available in the market that are specifically designed to communicate with your nervous system and send messages that are not being relayed through the usual means.

Relaxing Sun Exposure

This method of stimulation for the vagus nerve through sun exposure is still in the testing phase, but it has the potential to be acknowledged. Sunshine is a source of Vitamin D and improves mood, along with increasing energy level, supporting good sleep, lowering blood pressure, and preventing cancer.

For the vagal nerve, it is said to be beneficial through indirect means. The sun's rays are responsible for increasing the MSH (melanocyte-stimulating hormone) in the body, which is linked to increased vagal nerve activity. When we sit in the sun to bask, the body experiences vagal nerve stimulation indirectly.

You can pick any morning when the weather allows and spend it just taking in the sun. Think of it as a quick and short version of tanning.

5.1 Grounding Exercises

All vagus nerve-related exercises can be linked to the essence of grounding methods. These methods talk about how to divert your attention from external factors influencing your body to the internal factors that require your energy and effort.

There are a few exercises that can be considered calming and intuitive enough to guide your mind and body towards a good future. Use the exercises that are given ahead to keep focusing on making your ease of mind a priority above all else.

Practicing Meditation

Meditation is the most basic yet effective method for anyone to feel refreshed and calm even when stress gets over the mind and body. It can be very helpful to take some time and practice body scanning, which allows you to focus inwards.

In meditation, be mindful of your body by lying down and breathing deeply while noticing different body parts. Start with 5 minutes and increase the time gradually to 30 minutes.

One way to meditate is to start from top to bottom and breathe until you feel relieved.

Lighting a Scented Candle

Aromatherapy is one of the most invigorating exercises that not many people are familiar with. Take your time and consideration to find scented candles that smell soothing and relaxing to you.

Once you take your pick, spend ten minutes each day lighting the scented candle of your choice while meditating or breathing deeply.

Take a Bath

Taking a bath, especially a cold bath, can help you shock your body system into quickly working towards regulating itself. Any relaxing and grounding exercise that makes you jump allows the body to make an attempt to go back to its restive state.

The restive state can only be achieved once you take time to return to the normal routine. Taking a bath for 10 to 30 minutes can help you ground yourself after facing the stresses of daily life.

Use Distraction to Calm Down

Another way to ground yourself when struggling to do so is to look for things and activities that can serve as a distraction. For instance, if you feel that your heartbeat is too high and you cannot get yourself to calm down as you usually do, try taking deep breaths while looking, doing, or playing something relaxing.

If you feel relaxed by watching a comedy show or playing the guitar, it is best to take on any activity that you know can help. This way, you can ensure that your body doesn't lag behind and that you are able to keep up with it in the worst of times.

Make and Take Tea

Tea is a source of comfort. If you are too immersed in some thoughts that are making it difficult for you to shut off the brain, a good distraction method is to make and enjoy a cup of tea. By focusing on the task at hand, you are likely to put your worries aside and, in turn, regulate the body's function.

When you make tea, do not simply drink it. Pick the cup in your hands and feel the weight in your hands. Next, smell the soothing scent and take it in. Take small sips to savor the taste. Use mindfulness to bring peace to yourself.

You can also use this method with any other hot beverage as long as it qualifies as a comfort food to you.

Visualizing Happiness

Every person has one or more "happy places" where he or she can feel calm and comfortable. These places could be real or imaginary, but the happiness that one feels is absolutely real. If you are looking for ways to ground yourself after a tense situation, find and imagine things that bring you happiness (it will increase the vagal tone activity, too).

Your happy place could be any person, place, or object that brings you a sense of calm in highly chaotic situations. Whenever physical or mental pressures prove to be too much, use it as an escape route that brings you closer to solutions in a rational way.

Describing in Detail

Another way that is used for grounding yourself through distraction is to describe things around you in great detail. For example, you may have a lamp in your room, but when describing it in detail, you will note all of its features, such as its color, shape, design, height, width, closeness to you, contrast, or combination with the room as well as the environment it is in.

Take time to analyze your surroundings and give time to each object while describing their details. Whenever you find it hard to anchor yourself in reality, use this technique to stimulate your senses and bring your heart rate and blood pressure under control.

Play Mind Games

Grounding doesn't always need elaborate plans to work; a simple way of forgetting the issues that exacerbate your condition is to play games in your mind. Out of boredom, fun, or for a purpose, playing games can be the easiest way of finding something to do that forces the body to let go of the difficult things that plague your mind.

You can choose any game that comes to your mind. For example, spotting the car's lo, looking for letters while driving, or picking a random category and naming all items that fall under it. You can also start reciting something in an order or solve math equations. The possibilities are endless!

Following Music with a Pen

Another exercise that can prove fruitful for grounding yourself is to sit down with a piece of paper and a pen. Play any calming or soothing tune that you like. With music playing, start moving your pen with the rhythm, making abstract art as you go. Giving your whole attention to the music will help you become immersed in the beauty and serenity of music, actively making your body feel less hyper-alert and relaxed.

Sound Awareness

Sound awareness is an exercise that can be performed anywhere. All you need is to be in a comfortable position in your house, a park, or any other place that feels lively to you.

Be mindful of the sounds that fall on your ear; they could be the wind whistling through the window or the sound of children laughing and playing nearby. Start with the sounds that are being produced in your immediate vicinity and gradually listen to more distant sounds that need special concentration to be recognized.

This practice can be started with 2 minutes of your time initially before going up to 20 minutes. Pulling all your energies into listening can force the body to pay attention to slowing down the involuntary processes that are hard to steer otherwise.

CHAPTER 6

HEALTHY DIET FOR A HEALTHY LIFE

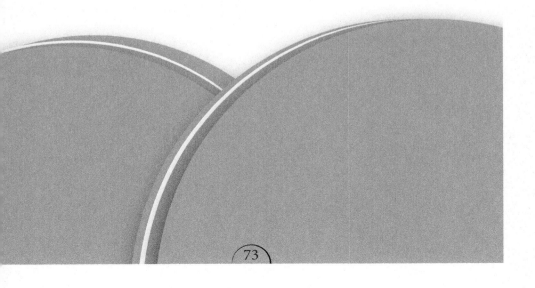

A healthy diet has been a trending topic in the past decade. People are becoming more conscious of their eating habits, and rightfully so, because good food allows us to stay sound physically and mentally for better outcomes.

Although it is true that not much research is being conducted on the connection between food and vagus nerves, as indirectly as it may be, the food that goes into our body affects every aspect of life and should be treated with the importance it deserves.

6.1 Focus on Gut-Health

We have already discussed the brain-gut axis for which the vagus nerve is responsible. The gut bacteria, as well as the neurons that are linked through this axis, need strength to perform bodily functions optimally.

The food we eat should be examined for nutrients and, specifically, the elements that are essential for the body in case of personal issues. For example, if a person suffers from a heart condition, his diet will vary from that of a healthy person with no apparent issues.

However, there are foods and nutrients that are necessary for all people who wish to keep their vagal nerve stimulated and in action. Another thing you can do to improve bodily functions is to take around three to five diaphragmatic breaths before each meal to stimulate the vagus nerve and aid digestion.

6.2 Foods to Include in Daily Routine

Food is one of the building blocks of your body. It is important to choose which foods and nutrients deserve your attention more than the others. Let's find out which food items you need to add or subtract from your life to promote healthy vagal nerve activity.

We will be focusing on foods that directly affect the vagus nerve and vagal tone of the body. Here are the details:

Probiotics

Probiotics are the live bacteria in fermented foods that are healthy to eat for humans. If you are a fan of foods such as yogurt, kimchi, kombucha, sauerkraut, and much more, you are already consuming bacteria that make your immunity better and your gut stronger.

Consuming fermented products allows the gut bacteria to flourish and perform well by activating the vagal nerve.

Omega-3 Fatty Acids

Omega-3 fatty acid is another essential nutrient of the body that regulates functions of the nervous system. Two main types of Omega-3 are DHA (docosahexaenoic acid) and

EPA (eicosapentaenoic acid); both are linked to critical functions of the vagus nerve, such as increasing heart rate variability and decreasing heart rate to its regular level.

Omega-3 is usually in abundance in fish and seafood of various kinds, but it can also be found in plant-based oils, seeds, nuts, tofu, brussels sprouts, and avocados.

Tryptophan Rich Foods

Tryptophan is an amino acid that plays a crucial role in maintaining metabolic functions of the body. It is also involved in the serotonin-making process that performs the mood-boosting functions in the body. It is also vital for astrocytes (the cells found in the brain and spinal cord) to perform well and control inflammation.

Tryptophan foods include nuts, seeds, spinach, bananas, pineapple, chickpeas, oats, red meat, fish, and poultry products.

High-Choline Foods

Choline is a nutrient that makes acetylcholine in the body, the main neurotransmitter that works for the parasympathetic system. In turn, it also affects the vagal tone. You should consume foods that contain choline to let the nervous system get its nutrients to keep working smoothly. The foods that are high in choline levels include red meat, eggs, fish, chicken, soybeans, kidney beans, cauliflower, red potatoes, shiitake mushrooms, and quinoa.

Although you should consume high-choline foods, it is advised not to go overboard because excessive intake can also cause other issues.

Sufficient Intake of Vitamin B

Another nutrient that is given importance these days and is linked to good vagal nerve health is vitamin B, more specifically, vitamin B12.

The neurotransmitters of the brain need a sufficient amount of vitamin B to keep working optimally. If you are running low on these, it is possible to feel numbness and pins and needles in various parts of the body.

You can add seeds, nuts, bananas, spinach, peaches, beans, poultry, dairy products, and eggs to your diet to increase vitamin B reserves in the body. Although there are a number of supplements available in the market for vitamin B, it is recommended to talk to a doctor before using them.

No to Sugar

Once you are sure that your vagus nerve needs intervention to heal or perform well, gradually cut the sugar from your life. I say gradually only because an immediate cut-off usually never works without intense motivation behind it.

Start by cutting the sugar intake in half and decreasing it daily. The reason for cutting sugar consumption is that the inflammation in or around the GI tract cannot be healed while you are still taking it. It causes chronic inflammation that also affects the signaling pathways that affect the gut-brain communication.

Fibrous Food

Eating foods that are rich in fiber can help the body to expel the waste regularly, thus reducing the likelihood of any problems in the intestines. A healthy GI tract will keep the inflammation and other risks at bay and maintain a healthy vagal tone.

Foods that are rich in fiber include beans, broccoli, whole grains, nuts, apples, avocados, berries, potatoes, and plain popcorn (made without butter or any other ingredient).

6.3 Intermittent Fasting

Intermittent fasting is said to have many benefits. It is said to aid all body functions, including heart rate regulation, support weight loss, boost metabolism rate, reduce inflammation, and increase insulin resistance in the body, among others.

Fasting aids in an increase in heart rate variability (HRV) that ensures an increase in parasympathetic activity as well as vagal tone.

Try it as a way to cleanse your body and mind by fasting for the larger part of the day. Start your practice by setting an achievable target before increasing time by one hour a day. An average fast could be 16 to 18 hours. But you can try reaching that level gradually.

You can also choose the frequency of fast-keeping for a week. For example, you can choose to fast once or twice a week on designated days to improve your physical health.

> **Did You Know?**
>
> Muslims keep fast in Islamic month of Ramadan. They keep consecutive fasts for the whole month where they do not eat or drink from sunrise to sunset.

Conclusion

The vagus nerve may not be an important organ or a function that people are hyper-focused on, but it doesn't remove the fact that it performs an essential function of the body. When you feel that your body cannot keep functioning as it is functioning now, it is best to look for reasons and then solutions.

Once you are familiar with what the vagus nerve is or what it does, it is best to implement the exercises, physical or mental, to eliminate the possibility of it becoming problematic for you.

Although we have offered many exercises in the book, I would urge you to try everything once and then select the ones that are useful to you alone. No treatment is always right for all patients, similarly, not all exercises will be popular hits either. Pick and choose the ones that prove to be beneficial to you.

About the Author

Queenie Dillon is a holistic health practitioner who has been providing home-based classes and guidance to private clients regarding their plans to achieve mental and physical health. She is focused on the topic of healing the body from the inside by improving the internal connection system of the body.

Dillon guides her students and clients to perform small exercises every day that can make them improve their vagal tone and many other bodily functions along the way.

Printed in Great Britain
by Amazon

46706541R00046